Jeramy Sianyang Durango Sanchez

Rehabilitation occupational therapy program

Jeramy Sianyang Durango Sanchez

Rehabilitation occupational therapy program

For older adults with epicondylitis

ScienciaScripts

Imprint

Any brand names and product names mentioned in this book are subject to trademark, brand or patent protection and are trademarks or registered trademarks of their respective holders. The use of brand names, product names, common names, trade names, product descriptions etc. even without a particular marking in this work is in no way to be construed to mean that such names may be regarded as unrestricted in respect of trademark and brand protection legislation and could thus be used by anyone.

Cover image: www.ingimage.com

This book is a translation from the original published under ISBN 978-620-2-14249-6.

Publisher:
Sciencia Scripts
is a trademark of
Dodo Books Indian Ocean Ltd. and OmniScriptum S.R.L publishing group

120 High Road, East Finchley, London, N2 9ED, United Kingdom
Str. Armeneasca 28/1, office 1, Chisinau MD-2012, Republic of Moldova, Europe
Printed at: see last page
ISBN: 978-620-6-86481-3

Table of Contents

SUMMARY

In the degree project, the pathology of acquired epicondylitis in older adults was presented at the Teodoro Maldonado Carbo Hospital, where they presented the condition obtained that limits older adults in their daily lives and in the work environment.

The objective of this research is the recovery of epicondylitis by means of physical agents such as thermotherapy, TENS and intervention plan through activities. The design of this research is descriptive and cross-sectional, since it reveals the reality of epicondylitis and its incidence in the work environment and household chores.

INTRODUCTION

The present work, which has as its theme REHABILITATION PROGRAM IN OCCUPATIONAL THERAPY FOR USERS WITH EPICONDYLITIS IN OLDER ADULTS, aims to create a rehabilitation program with exercises and therapeutic methods that include cryotherapy, ultrasound, electrodes and, therefore, the pathology called epicondylitis.

Epicondylitis is a common pathology suffered by adults or athletes, who performed repetitive movements, both work and sport, it is a pathology that degenerates the tendon, 90% of people have improvement to conservative treatment, and in some very severe cases, recovery is surgical.(1)

The frequency of this pathology results in injuries due to overloaded movements affecting the extensor muscles located in the forearm, producing tears and causing limitations in the user's movements, making him/her a dependent person.(2)

To give an accurate diagnosis in this pathology that affects the elbow in older adults, we must develop a clinical history, such as their profession, dominance, their daily activities that can produce this pathology, getting to complete the information that will help us to know why epicondylitis was produced in this patient.(3)

Taking into account that epicondylitis is caused by repetitive movements, such as exerting some load at work or tennis sport, which degenerates this pathology, which in a period of time comes to atrophy the elbow joint. The aforementioned topic was selected because of an interest to improve the functionality of people suffering from this pathology, since most of the population has it, however they do not show importance, thinking that it is a common pain, aggravating the situation.

Epicondylitis, which causes affliction in the epicondyle area, produces weakness in the action of the extension movement, showing a slight delay in muscle contraction, produces a decrease in the range of mobilization of the elbow area, and also decreases the strength at the time of the action of wanting to grasp light or heavy objects.(4)

I personally chose this research topic, since most people with this pathology, live thinking that it is a pain or limitation of normal movement caused by age or sport, worsening their way of life in the long term, without being treated or performing any type of rehabilitative treatment.

Chapter 1 discusses the symptoms of epicondylitis, as well as the disadvantages it can cause at work and in daily life activities, decreasing your independence and seriously affecting the muscles and tendons in the forearm that help extend the fingers.

In most people the symptom or pathology lasts between 9 to 12 months, in some cases in people without proper treatment, can be extended, so they must perform a rehabilitation plan to improve the injury, some effective treatments are therapeutic activities, or implementation of compresses or shock waves. (5)

One therapeutic method is shock waves, since it is non-invasive, and is tolerated by most patients without side effects, the objective of this method is to assess the effectiveness, and improve the pain of the affected area in this case the elbow, helping to increase joint range. (6)

Another beneficial method for older users with epicondylitis, are the TENS, which are the cause of giving a transcutaneous electrical stimulation that serves to relieve pain, this is a small device usually portable, which emits small electrical pulses in a gentle and totally safe way that mostly neutralizes the pain.

TENS produces analgesia, which will help the patient to perform in a correct and painless way the activities that the therapist will propose, helping the physical improvement, caused by pain and weakness in the upper extremities that limit the activities of daily living.

It is advisable to use TENS in this case, for epicondylitis, it is beneficial to use them, knowing in which place they should be placed, the time in case of acute pain, you can apply them from 15 to 20 minutes, in cases of chronic pain can be applied up to 30 minutes.

The benefits of using this type of method, called TENS in epicondylitis, is to relieve pain almost immediately, also ensures muscle relief, this type of therapy is available at home because it is completely safe, it is recommended to perform at least 10 sessions with this type of therapy.

By performing the program of therapeutic exercises and implementation of compresses which will help relieve pain and inflammation caused by epicondylitis, also improve the articular range of the elbow. Cryotherapy has several benefits such as analgesic and anti-inflammatory effects, which help to reduce and prevent tissue inflammation. Not only tennis professionals suffer or acquire this pathology since it is called "tennis elbow" is also acquired by workers such as those who work in warehouses, which perform the same movements in arms and with considerable weight.

Among the symptoms of epicondylitis we find pain that starts from the outside of the elbow to the forearm in the action of grasping objects or with the pronosupination movement, in a few cases there may be a symptom of weakness at the time of grasping objects, in severe cases there is noticeable inflammation along with reduced mobility.

In epicondylitis the most serious impediment is pain, which causes weakness and hinders the activities of daily living in the older adult, the most used method in epicondylitis is conservative, rehabilitative, as a last option surgery will be taken into account, when this pathology has advanced considerably.(7)

The age of this condition is between the fifth and sixth decade of life, the diagnosis is characterized mainly by localized pain in the elbow in the lateral area, and decreased strength at the time of grip, decreased range of mobility and altered functions of the upper extremities. (8)

People suffering from tennis elbow can alleviate pain by the therapeutic method with electrodes, since it can be used as an analgesic method, to increase efficiency and improvement, this method should be accompanied by a rehabilitation program of exercises achieving a high degree of effectiveness. (9)

CHAPTER I

THE PROBLEM

1.1.   PROBLEM STATEMENT

Epicondylitis is a common pathology of the elbow, it is produced by an excessive use of the extensor muscles of the forearm, performed by athletes or workers. It produces pain in the sides of the elbow, also produces loss of strength and rarely generates disability. The symptoms are usually long lasting, normally from 6 to 9 months, there are surgical, medical and rehabilitative treatments where we will find the use of cryotherapy with ultrasound and electrodes.

The tennis elbow called epicondylitis is worldwide where, first world countries in this case America, are treated with a specialist correctly, in another point of view, in South America is at least 70% in which people with epicondylitis are attended by a professional, generalizing, in Ecuador, where the highest percentage of people suffer from the pathology think it is a common pain coming to take just ordinary drugs to treat it.

The cause of epicondylitis is caused by overuse of the joint, which is the repetitive movement of the muscles found in the forearm where it is used to extend or lift the hand, this type of repetitive motion that causes wear and tear, can cause from a minor injury to very small tears as a bony prominence on the outside of the elbow.

The risk factors that influence this pathology increase when some characteristics are present, such as age, where it is more frequent to acquire it from 30 to 60 years old, also included is the occupation where repetitive movements are performed in the work, at this point is the sport, where repetitive movements and an overload are performed.

Epicondylitis, very common in older people who have complications as time goes by, where the muscles or tendons of the elbow degenerate or atrophy, therefore, a rehabilitation treatment program will be carried out, including occupational activities and implementation of cryotherapy and electrodes.

The condition called epicondylitis causes pain, producing a disability in the functions of daily life, causing problems both labor and sports problems. Epicondylitis is acquired at the age of 35 to 60 years, most users respond to rehabilitation treatment, there are very few cases in which patients do not see results from the rehabilitation plan, which leads to surgery.

The aim of this work is to strengthen or increase the user's range of mobility, disappear the pain and increase dependence, developing activities that will help him to carry out daily life activities, where he can assert himself, and demonstrating that epicondylitis is not just a common pain, but a pathology that, over time, can degenerate the joint.

1.2.   PROBLEM FORMULATION

What influence does the application of the occupational rehabilitation program have on patients with epicondylitis?

1.3.   JUSTIFICATION AND IMPORTANCE:

In view of the problems identified, this research focuses on identifying the percentage of older adults with epicondylitis problems, and the influence of the rehabilitation program, directed from occupational therapy to ensure the quality of life of this population. It should be noted that, in his work, the occupational therapist integrates the program together with compresses to maintain good health and prevent the deterioration of functions in older adults as a result of epicondylitis.

Based on the above, through this therapeutic plan we will be able to introduce healthy habits or activities in order to improve physical condition, reduce limitations, strengthen muscles, improve range of motion, joint amplitude, balance and coordination of older adults in the Teodoro Maldonado Carbo Hospital. Thus providing them with the ability to achieve greater independence, so they can have a good quality of life.

The development of this work will provide evidence on the benefits of the therapeutic program in epicondylitis, data that will allow not only to expand professional practice, but also therapeutic strategies used for the group studied in terms of autonomy, well-being and independence.

The elderly will benefit the most, since they are the most prone to accidents and in some cases they live alone, therefore, they will benefit from the rehabilitation plan, thus improving their daily life activities or in some cases improving their work activities.

The usefulness of the rehabilitation plan is for adults, such as workers or athletes, to maintain their motor skills to the maximum without any limitation, to live in a pleasant way, and also to keep people informed that epicondylitis is not only a common pain, but a condition that can become a major physical limitation.

The important contributions of this research is to obtain a good lifestyle without complications, limited in the upper limb, which is very important to be able to be an independent person, since many people who have been treated managed to overcome this condition.

1.4.   GENERAL AND SPECIFIC OBJECTIVES:

1.4.1. General Objective

To strengthen or increase range of motion through the application of an occupational rehabilitation program for older adults with epicondylitis.

1.4.2. Specific Objectives

- **Identify what type of limitations are present in the population in order to intervene with a therapeutic plan.**
- **Strengthen physical skills during daily movements and thus perform therapeutic activities.**

- **Integrate participatory exercise routines to promote healthy activities by relieving pain and increasing movement.**

1.5.   DELIMITATION OF THE RESEARCH:

Field of study: Health.

Area of research: Occupational Therapy.

Aspects: Enabler.

Time: April to July 2023.

Subject: OCCUPATIONAL THERAPY REHABILITATION PROGRAM FOR USERS WITH EPICONDYLITIS IN OLDER ADULTS.

Venue: Teodoro Maldonado Carbo.

Line of research: Human and animal health.

Sublines of research: Diagnostic and therapeutic, biological, biochemical and molecular methodologies.

Subject of study: Older adults with mobility problems.

1.6.   FEASIBILITY AND VIABILITY OF THE RESEARCH:

Feasibility

This case or research is considered feasible because we have the availability of the population and access to the environment where it will be performed. Where there are several clinical and hospital institutions where we can find people suffering from this pathology, the research will be conducted with the consent of the patient and hospital, which will be in an ethical manner.

Feasibility.

It is considered feasible since the resources are available to carry out the research, having in the area a professional team specialized in the field of occupational therapy. It also provides access to the required population and to the instruments for the evaluation.

CHAPTER II

THEORETICAL FRAME

2.1   BACKGROUND

The research carried out by Alberto, 2022 which had as title "Tennis elbow epicondylitis)" whose objective was to comment that epicondylitis is the pathology of the elbow, produced when performing repetitive movements, for which, it is common that adult people who practiced tennis or any other sport, including some type of work that includes repetitive movements, cause this type of pathology. This results in the forearm muscles and tendons atrophy due to overuse, repeating movements as in sports or workers, affecting in the long term, causing in people a feeling of distress, along with sensitivity located in the affected area.(10)

The research carried out by Ramírez Salvany, 2022 which was entitled "Physiotherapeutic treatment of epicondylitis" aimed to demonstrate the effectiveness of physiotherapeutic treatment for the improvement and recovery of people with this condition, reducing pain and increasing the functionality of the joint. The methodology was selected by searching in different data banks, obtaining these are obtained by including discernment. The results show that the Mulligan technique has very significant benefits to the decrease of pain. (11)

The research carried out by Planas Lara, 2021 that had as title "Aplicativo de ayuda para la valoración de la epicondilitis profesional" has as objective the tool to check or identify which specific tasks have a high probability of generating this pathology, which allows in the case of work, professional older adults, to have an ergonomic area to avoid epicondylitis. The methodology is the ergonomic normative that is focused on the biomechanics of the elbow proving to be more specific than other methods. The result is the effective demonstration that determines professional contingencies that are able to identify epicondylitis pathologies. (12)

2.2 THEORETICAL BACKGROUND

Occupational therapy

Occupational therapy is about activities of therapeutic use of care, play, leisure or work, which is responsible for maximizing the independence of the person, maximize the development and to prevent some kind of disability, which may include some adaptation in the environment and improve the quality of life of the patient.

Definition of occupational therapy

It is a promotion of health and well-being through occupations, the objective of which is to enable patients to intervene in the activities of daily living. Thus providing daily programs to maximize their independence and self-reliance.

Importance of occupational therapy

It is important because it benefits the person to improve their quality of life when affected by any pathology, disease or disability. It can help people learn personal care or grooming skills, improve range of motion, maximize capacity for activities of daily living.

Occupational therapy is important because it assesses the degree of independence, helps to enhance daily living skills and functions in general, evaluates both the physical and psychosocial aspects of the patient according to the therapist's plan.

Occupational therapy approach

This therapy has a humanistic approach that includes kindness and a plan or regimen in the patient's daily life that includes creative activities or occupations, which is focused on people who suffer from some type of illness or disability, either physical or cognitive.

One of the approaches is to convert adaptations for children or adults, to perform a specific task, who is in a situation of vulnerability, helping through a plan to convert their environment into adaptations and become someone independent.

Epicondylitis

Definition of epicondylitis

This condition called epicondylitis is the most common, since it is the tendon degeneration of the elbow, which impacts workers who perform repetitive movements of pronation or extension of the forearm and hand, such as professionals who use tools like hammers.

Epicondylitis is a tendon disorder that causes pain, limiting a functional physical limitation. It also occurs in older adults due to some type of work or sport that includes repetitive movements, which puts the epicondyle tendon at risk.

Etiology of epicondylitis

This pathology is caused by performing tasks that lead to repetition movements and poor posture of the upper limb, this type of tasks in older adults produce pathologies in the tendon, which is triggered by repetition movements, performing hand extension and pronation of the forearm. (13)

Classification of epicondylitis

Epicondylitis is divided or classified into three parts, the first is mild, also called tendinosis, which affects 20% of the tendon, the second is moderate, where there may be a tear in the tendon between 20% to 80% and finally we find the severe where there is a total tear of the tendon.

Diagnosis of epicondylitis

It is based on a medical or clinical history and a physical examination, in most of the people who present this condition it is treated with a conservative plan, mainly with the decrease of the activity that gave birth to this pathology, helping to correct the abnormalities of this.

Rehabilitation programs

TENS

This method called TENS is the application of the technique of transcutaneous electrical nerve stimulation, and this produces an analgesic effect, can also reduce pain from the first session, positively influences muscle activity in patients with motor pathologies.

This is a small device that can be portable, battery operated or directly connected, emits electricity in a gentle and totally safe way that helps relieve pain, also known as electrodes, which include adhesive patches placed on the skin.

This device called TENS produces electrical impulses that do not cause pain that goes to the nervous system, the placement of this varies according to its location of the pathology, also varies its intensity graduation that will be the most convenient for the patient.

TENS helps to considerably decrease the pain in the area affected by epicondylitis, and helps to increase the pressure force, this produces an analgesia that releases or activates the neurotransmitters involved in inhibiting pain, helping to perform the therapy.(14)

Regarding the increase in pressure strength achieved by patients with epicondylitis after completing the treatment, one explanation for the improvement is the analgesia produced by TENS, since in the rehabilitation process it helped to perform activities in the forearm, strengthening the muscular part of the forearm (14).(14)

Thermotherapy in epicondylitis

The objective of thermotherapy is to treat the pain and inflammation produced in the elbow, in order to achieve functional recovery of the upper limb, to be able to carry out their work again, without any limitation both painful and sensitive.

This type of therapy helps to reduce muscle spasms and stiffness, also in reducing pain, is applied in an estimated 20 to 30 minutes in the affected area, with a temperature less than 40 ° C, is applied by hot or warm compresses.

The indicated temperature of thermotherapy should always be higher than the user's temperature, i.e. higher than 37°C, and not higher than 40°C, since it will not be beneficial above this temperature, it also depends on the patient and his sensitivity, it is indicated to apply it at least 3 times a day.

Therapeutic exercise

This will be applied as routines or physical training that will be to promote good health, these types of exercises will improve grip strength as well as range of motion, it will also help to tone muscles by relieving stiffness, a program should be made to meet the needs of the user.

Among the exercises performed by the patient, will help in physical improvement, improving forearm flexion, forearm extension, pronation and supination. These types of exercises will help the flexibility of the affected arm, to be able to perform their personal activities.

Among the exercises performed, we have to improve the extension, with the help of a support on the elbow, and firmly grasping with the hand a cylinder, it is proposed to perform the pronosupination movement, trying to fulfill the full range of motion.

For the improvement of wrist flexion, to increase flexion, we must perform the following activity, placing the forearm on a wide and flat support, leaving the hand hanging on the edge, with the palmar side up, the next step is to place a weight of 1 or 2 pounds, lifting the wrist in a slow way, without lifting the forearm off the table, repeating the movement 8 to 12 times, in series of 3, repeating the exercise with the palm down.

Exercise to maximize biceps flexion you have to sit in an inclined manner, with the hand resting on the thigh, resting the elbow of the other hand on the thigh holding a dumbbell, slowly flexing the arm, lifting the dumbbell towards the chest part, repeating 8 to 12 times in sets of 3.

To increase grip strength, we can hold a stress ball or a rolled up sock, pressing on the object, keeping it pressed for 5 seconds, repeating 8 to 12 times, recommended 3 to 5 times a day.

To increase the resistance, we must place ourselves on a chair with our back straight supported to the chair, raising the elbow next to the arm in a straight way, extending it fully to chest level, closing the hand with force for 5 seconds, noticing improvement will be added weight of max. 2 pounds.

To correct the radial deviation caused by epicondylitis, with the help of an elastic band, place the arm on a flat surface and the hand in neutral position, deflecting it towards the top in a time of 5 seconds each repetition, this exercise will have 5 repetitions and 3 series.

In the increase of the supination movement, with the help of an elastic band or resistance band, with the forearm slightly flexed, place the band on the palm, making resistance with the other hand, making the supination movement maintaining the movements 5 seconds, 5 repetitions and 3 series.

To strengthen pronation, with the help of an elastic band held with the opposite hand, leaning on a table, rotate the forearm and palm down, making the pronation, in repetitions of 5 and series of 3, each movement should last 5 seconds.

Performing an exercise to promote epicondylar stretching, we must extend several arms at chest height, palms down, one on top of the other, helping to flex the arm with epicondylitis to the maximum, until a feeling of tension and maintain this position for 30 seconds.

2.3   CONCEPTUAL FRAMEWORK

Epicondylitis: Epicondylitis is a degenerative pathology in the tendon area, most patients respond positively to conservative treatment, in those who do not see results, which are few, surgery is recommended.(15)

Characteristic: This condition is highly related to work or athletes, being very frequent in the population, usually acquired by people whose age is between 40 and 55 years, is characterized by the presence of pain and decreased grip strength.(8)

Affectation: Tennis elbow affects the muscles located in the epicondyle, it is listed as a condition with a higher incidence rate in the workplace, where people suffer from it without realizing it, this pathology affects the performance of skills used in daily life.(16)

Treatment: The ideas required to treat this condition that most adults suffer from, thinking that it is a normal pain, is treated with an intervention plan programmed for each patient, such as rehabilitative exercises or application of agents such as TENS.

In the case of rehabilitative exercises, they are recommended because they help to strengthen or increase the lost joint range, and increase grip strength, this also helps us to relieve pain and regain the independence of the person affected by epicondylitis.

Compress: By means of hot compresses, it helps us to deflate the affected area together with vasodilatation, this method also helps us to relieve the pain in the elbow, helping to perform in a correct way the conservative treatment given by the therapist.

TENS: With the help of the TENS application method, these reduce the activity of the cells that cause pain, causing muscular relief and reduction of stiffness in the affected area, by means of small electrical impulses that are modulated by the therapist.

2.4   LEGAL FRAMEWORK

Organic Law for the Elderly

Art. 16.- Right to a dignified life. To guarantee the integral protection that the State, society and family must provide to older adults, with the purpose of achieving the effective enjoyment of their rights, duties and responsibilities; they shall have the right to access to resources and opportunities for work, economic, political, educational, cultural, spiritual and recreational activities, as well as the improvement of their skills, competencies and potentialities, to achieve their personal and community development that will allow them to promote their personal autonomy.

Art. 7.- Every person, without discrimination for any reason whatsoever, has the following rights in relation to health: a) Universal, equitable, permanent, timely and quality access to all health actions and services.

Art. 42.-The right to integral health. The State shall guarantee older adults the right without discrimination to physical, mental, sexual and reproductive health and shall ensure universal, supportive, equitable and timely access to promotion, prevention, recovery, rehabilitation, palliative, priority, functional and comprehensive care services, in the entities that make up the National Health System, with a gender, generational and intercultural approach.

2.5   OPERATIONALIZATION OF VARIABLES

Tabla 1.   Operationalization of variables

Variable	Operational definition	Dimension	Indicator	Source

Older adult.	Adults over 60 years of age.	Limitations of physical abilities.	60 - 85 years.	Interview.
Rehabilitation program.	Exercise plan and placement of agents to relieve pain and improve motor skills lost due to epicondylitis.	Decrease in pain.	0 = no pain 10 = Maximum pain.	Primary source.
Epicondylitis	Tendinous degeneration of the elbow	Slight moderate	Relative frequency	Medical history

CHAPTER III

METHODOLOGICAL FRAMEWORK

3.1 FOCUS

The approach of the present work is qualitative because it is based on data collection to test a certain hypothesis and a statistical analysis to form a pattern of behavior. It is qualitative because it chooses a certain idea, which formulates several totally important research questions, after doing this, it develops the hypothesis and variables, along with a plan to test them, measuring the variables and analyzing the measurements obtained.

In short, the quantitative research approach is one that is based on the collection and analysis of numerical data in order to describe or predict such pathologies. In this case, epicondylitis, the quantitative approach will be used to determine what type of rehabilitation plan to use.

3.2 TYPE AND DESIGN OF RESEARCH

This research is cross-sectional since it was carried out in an established field period in addition to being observational.

3.2.1 Design types

The type of design that will be used in the study on epicondylitis is descriptive, since it is a type of research that has as its main objective to document the attitudes or characteristic of that population.

3.3 RESEARCH LEVELS

3.3.1 Descriptive level

The descriptive type of research is used to gather information or data on the variables to which they refer, either collectively or individually. The purpose of this descriptive level is to identify the profile traits of the person or groups of people, collecting information for the object of analysis.

3.4   PERIOD AND PLACE WHERE THE RESEARCH IS CARRIED OUT

Time: May to July (8 weeks)

Location: Teodoro Maldonado Carbo

Located on 25 de Julio Avenue

Ecuador - Guayas - Guayaquil

3.5   POPULATION AND SAMPLE

3.5.1 Population

The population is a particular group of people found in a city or establishment, who have data such as age, sex, race or a special common goal whose interest is the same, can be quite broad. (17)

The population is determined by 15 patients with a diagnosis of epicondylitis.

3.5.2 Sample

The sample is the people selected from the population that is used for the study, to obtain information and conclusions in a valid way, this must be selected in an adequate way to guarantee the validity of the results obtained.

Sample: 20 adults between 60 and 65 years of age.

3.5.2.1   Sample calculation

A non-probabilistic random sample was used to calculate the sample to which the exclusion and inclusion criteria were applied in order to obtain a pure sample with which we can carry out this degree work.

3.5.2.2   Sampling

These samples refer to the non-probabilistic type, since the patients selected depend on meeting certain criteria or characteristics in order to fit into the research, so that the degree work can be carried out accurately.

3.5.2.3   Inclusion criteria

- Age: Adults should be between 60 to 85 years old, as the therapeutic treatment caused by epicondylitis is specifically focused on that age range, where treatment plays a crucial role in recovery.
- Motor difficulties: The adult should have some limitation of the upper extremity, including pain, numbness, sensation of weakness or decreased grip strength.
- Person with mild and moderate epicondylitis.
- People who agreed to be part of the project.

3.5.2.4   Exclusion criteria

- Dependents: Adults who can fend for themselves, without some type of pathology or pain on movement.
- Persons who did not consent to participate in the study.
- People with severe epicondylitis.

3.6   DATA COLLECTION TECHNIQUES AND INSTRUMENTS

The techniques implemented in this rehabilitation plan were therapeutic exercises and application of TENS in the affected area for the improvement of the patient with mild and moderate lateral epicondylitis in older adults with limitations in their activities of daily living.

The data acquired were from medical records obtained from the Teodoro Maldonado Carbo hospital, which helped with patient information, such as age, pathology or even the person's occupation, which will help develop the rehabilitation plan.

To obtain more data about the patient, such as limitations and pain, we apply two methods or interviews that will help in the development, which are the Barthel index and the tennis elbow test.

3.7   ETHICAL ASPECTS

The ethical considerations that are based on the area to the people who were taken as patients, where it is indicated how important it is to explain the consent or give approval to be subjects of the degree work where in a document it is communicated that they will be part of such work, who give in advance the approval in written form.

Approval and acceptance of the TEODORO MALDONADO CARBO hospital to allow the completion of the degree project on epicondylitis in older adults.

3.8   STATISTICAL ANALYSIS

This analysis will be directed to the collection of information or data based on the clinical histories of those patients with epicondylitis who are in the Teodoro Maldonado Carbo, who are within the inclusion criteria.

These data will be transferred in a Microsoft Excel sheet with the objective in order to put in order all the data obtained from the patient.

A statistical analysis will be prepared for qualitative variables with presentation of absolute values.

CHAPTER IV

RESULTS AND DISCUSSION

The following chapter reports the results obtained from the patients who were used for the present investigation.

4.1   RESULTS

Characteristics of the population

⬇ Genre

Tabla 2.   Gender distribution of patients with elbow epicondylitis

SEX	FREQUENCY	PERCENTAGE
Female	10,0	67%
Male	5,0	33%
TOTAL	15,0	100%

Source: Patient information sheet

Prepared by: Jeramy Durango (2023)

Gráfico 1. Gender distribution of patients with elbow epicondylitis

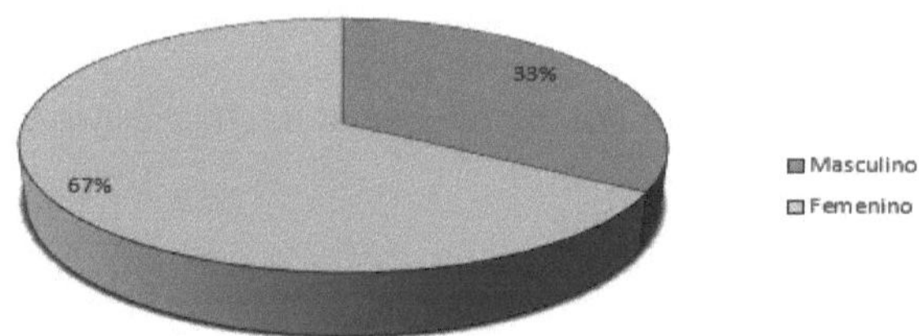

Source: Patient information sheet

Prepared by: Jeramy Durango (2023)

Analysis and interpretation

Of the total of 15 patients with elbow epicondylitis who participated in the study, 10 users were female, while 5 were male, i.e. 67% of the patients were female and 33% of the patients who participated were male.

🞣 Age range

Tabla 3. Age distribution of patients with epicondylitis of the elbow

	FREQUENCY	PERCENTAGE
60 - 64	4,0	27%
65 - 70	7,0	46%
71 - 76	3,0	20%
77 - 82	1,0	7%
TOTAL	15,0	100%

Source: Patient information sheet

Prepared by: Jeramy Durango (2023)

Gráfico 2. Age distribution of patients with epicondylitis of the elbow

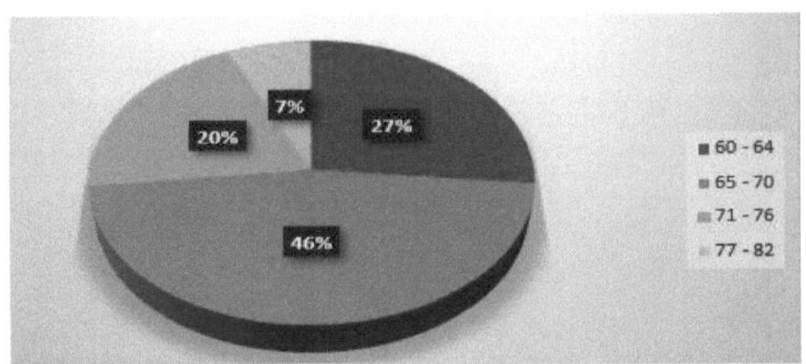

Source: Patient information sheet

Prepared by: Jeramy Durango (2023)

Analysis and interpretation

A total of 15 patients with elbow epicondylitis participated in the present study, with ages ranging from 60 to 82 years old, thus obtaining a total of 100% of the population studied. There are 7 older adults in an interval of 65 - 70 years corresponding to 46%, 4 older adults in an interval of 60 - 64 years corresponding to 27%, in an interval of 71 - 76 years there are 3 patients corresponding to 20%

and in an interval of 77 - 82 years there is 1 patient corresponding to 7% of the population with epicondylitis of the elbow studied.

⁍ Elbow affected by epicondylitis

Tabla 4. Distribution by affected elbow in patients with epicondylitis

AFFECTED ELBOW	NO. OF PATIENTS
Right elbow	12,0
Left elbow	3,0
Total	15,0

Source: Patient information sheet

Prepared by: Jeramy Durango (2023)

Gráfico 3. Distribution by elbow affected in patients with epicondylitis

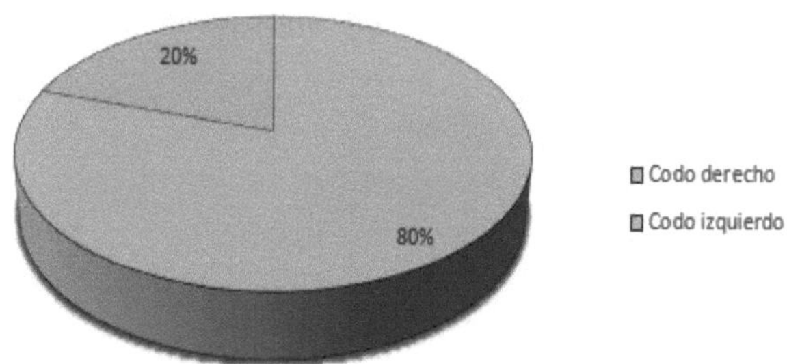

Source: Patient information sheet

Prepared by: Jeramy Durango (2023)

Analysis and interpretation

When a study was made to observe which elbow was affected, it was obtained that, of the total of 15 patients used for the present investigation, 12 of them had an epicondylitis condition in the right elbow, which corresponds to 80% of the total number of patients, while 3 patients had an epicondylitis condition in the left elbow, which represents 20% of the patients who were needed for the investigation.

Results of the assessment tests

⬥ Level of functional independence

Tabla 5.   Barthel Index

DEGREE OF INDEPENDENCE	SCORING	INITIAL EVALUATION	INITIAL RESULT	FINAL EVALUATION	FINAL RESULT
Total Dependence	0 - 20	0,0	0%	0,0	0%
Severe Dependency	20 - 35	0,0	0%	0,0	0%
Moderate Dependence	40 - 55	2,0	13%	1,0	7%
Mild Dependency	60 - 95	13,0	87%	9,0	60%
Independence	100	0,0	0%	5,0	33%
TOTAL		15,0	100%	15,0	100%

Source: Patient information sheet

Prepared by: Jeramy Durango (2023)

Gráfico 4. Barthel Index

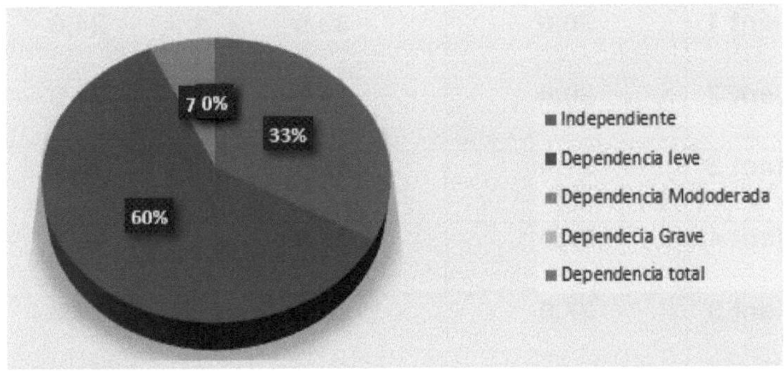

Source: Patient information sheet
Prepared by: Jeramy Durango (2023)

Analysis and interpretation

In this graph, it is possible to notice the improvement obtained by the users with respect to the initial evaluation. The evaluation was carried out using the Barthel Index to measure the degree of functional dependence of the patients when performing basic activities of daily living. 9 patients showed results of mild dependence giving a percentage result of 60%, 5 users went from mild dependence to independence to perform their activities of daily living giving a result of 33%, while 1 user remained in moderate dependence giving as a result 7% of the population studied.

↓ Degree of pain intensity, functional impairment and activities of daily living

Tabla 6.   Epicondylitis test score evaluated by user

PATIENT NO.	PAIN IN YOUR AFFECTED ARM	FUNCTIONAL DISORDER	DAILY ACTIVITIES
Patient 1	30,0	33,0	24,0
Patient 2	30,0	33,0	24,0
Patient 3	31,0	42,0	28,0
Patient 4	27,0	31,0	26,0
Patient 5	27,0	36,0	24,0

Patient 6	37,0	34,0	27,0
Patient 7	26,0	31,0	23,0
Patient 8	26,0	31,0	23,0
Patient 9	31,0	31,0	24,0
Patient 10	32,0	29,0	25,0
Patient 11	30,0	31,0	28,0
Patient 12	24,0	28,0	22,0
Patient 13	28,0	27,0	23,0
Patient 14	28,0	28,0	23,0
Patient 15	35,0	42,0	32,0

Source: Patient information sheet

Prepared by: Jeramy Durango (2023)

Gráfico 5. Score Epicondylitis test evaluated by user

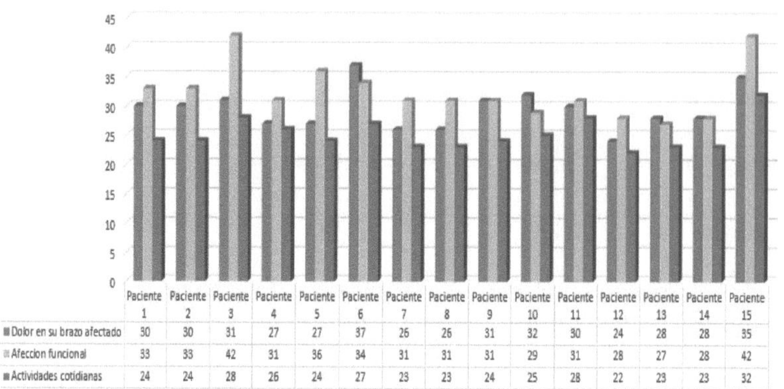

	Paciente 1	Paciente 2	Paciente 3	Paciente 4	Paciente 5	Paciente 6	Paciente 7	Paciente 8	Paciente 9	Paciente 10	Paciente 11	Paciente 12	Paciente 13	Paciente 14	Paciente 15
Dolor en su brazo afectado	30	30	31	27	27	37	26	26	31	32	30	24	28	28	35
Afeccion funcional	33	33	42	31	36	34	31	31	31	29	31	28	27	28	42
Actividades cotidianas	24	24	28	26	24	27	23	23	24	25	28	22	23	23	32

Source: Patient information sheet

Prepared by: Jeramy Durango (2023)

Analysis and interpretation

During the investigation, use was made of the epicondylitis test, in order to correctly analyze and understand the evaluation and reevaluation results, it should be taken into account that the areas between 0 - 10 points are evaluated, where 0 represents the minimum pain and difficulty in performing activities of daily living and 10 represents the maximum pain and difficulty in performing activities of daily living. The results of the user-rated epicondylitis test are presented, obtained from each user that was needed within the research, the evaluation and data collection was performed within each area found in the Patient-Rated Tennis Elbow Test (PRTEE), where it was obtained that within the area "pain in your affected arm"; the scores ranged between 26 - 37 points, in the area of "functional affection" the scores ranged between 27 - 42 points and in the area "daily activities" the scores ranged between 22 - 28 points.

⬥ Degree of pain in the affected arm (initial assessment - final assessment)

Tabla 7.   User-assessed epicondylitis test score - affliction in affected arm

PATIENT NO.	PAIN IN YOUR AFFECTED ARM	
	INITIAL EVALUATION	FINAL EVALUATION
Patient 1	30,0	7,0
Patient 2	30,0	7,0
Patient 3	31,0	4,0
Patient 4	27,0	7,0
Patient 5	27,0	12,0
Patient 6	37,0	7,0
Patient 7	26,0	10,0
Patient 8	26,0	10,0
Patient 9	31,0	7,0
Patient 10	32,0	14,0
Patient 11	30,0	13,0
Patient 12	24,0	11,0
Patient 13	28,0	15,0
Patient 14	28,0	7,0
Patient 15	35,0	14,0

Source: Patient information sheet
Prepared by: Jeramy Durango (2023)

Gráfico 6. User-assessed epicondylitis test score - affliction in affected arm

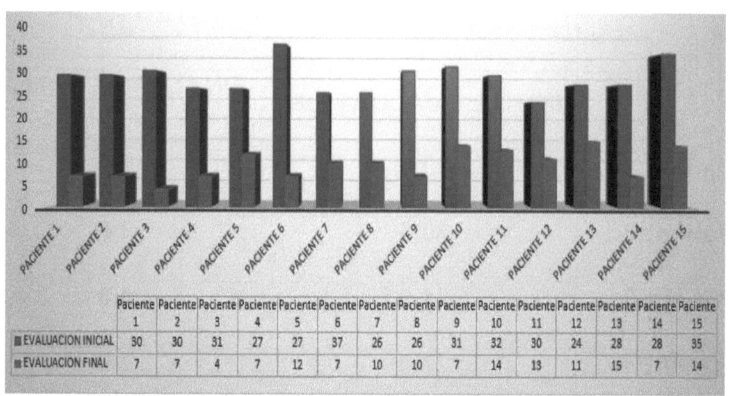

	Paciente 1	Paciente 2	Paciente 3	Paciente 4	Paciente 5	Paciente 6	Paciente 7	Paciente 8	Paciente 9	Paciente 10	Paciente 11	Paciente 12	Paciente 13	Paciente 14	Paciente 15
EVALUACION INICIAL	30	30	31	27	27	37	26	26	31	32	30	24	28	28	35
EVALUACION FINAL	7	7	4	7	12	7	10	10	7	14	13	11	15	7	14

Source: Patient information sheet

Prepared by: Jeramy Durango (2023)

Analysis and interpretation

During the investigation, use was made of the user-assessed epicondylitis test, the initial evaluation and a subsequent reevaluation were performed, where we can note a considerable improvement in users affected by elbow epicondylitis, it can be seen that the total results in the area of "pain in the affected arm" during the initial evaluation ranged between 24 - 35 where they had results of medium pain and unbearable pain when moving the affected arm, After the intervention, the results were obtained by applying a re-evaluation, where a notable improvement can be observed, where the results oscillate between 4 - 15 points, giving a notable improvement of 20 total points with respect to the initial interval and the final interval of the evaluation.

⬥ Degree of functional impairment (initial assessment - final assessment)

PATIENT NO.	FUNCTIONAL DISORDER	
	INITIAL EVALUATION	FINAL EVALUATION
Patient 1	33,0	6,0
Patient 2	33,0	6,0
Patient 3	42,0	5,0
Patient 4	31,0	7,0
Patient 5	36,0	7,0
Patient 6	34,0	11,0
Patient 7	31,0	8,0
Patient 8	31,0	8,0
Patient 9	31,0	10,0
Patient 10	29,0	10,0
Patient 11	31,0	11,0
Patient 12	28,0	10,0
Patient 13	27,0	11,0
Patient 14	28,0	8,0
Patient 15	42,0	10,0

Source: Patient information sheet

Prepared by: Jeramy Durango (2023)

Gráfico 7. User-assessed epicondylitis elbow test score - Functional condition

	Paciente 1	Paciente 2	Paciente 3	Paciente 4	Paciente 5	Paciente 6	Paciente 7	Paciente 8	Paciente 9	Paciente 10	Paciente 11	Paciente 12	Paciente 13	Paciente 14	Paciente 15
EVALUACION INICIAL	33	33	42	31	36	34	31	31	31	29	31	28	27	28	42
EVALUACION FINAL	6	6	5	7	7	11	8	8	10	10	11	10	11	8	10

Source: Patient information sheet
Prepared by: Jeramy Durango (2023)

Analysis and interpretation

During the present investigation in which the user-assessed epicondylitis test was used, an initial evaluation and a subsequent re-evaluation were performed, in which improvement can be noted in users affected by elbow epicondylitis in the area of "functional affection", it can be noted that during the initial evaluation the scores ranged between 27 - 42 where the results showed that patients had medium difficulty, severe and even inability to perform activities requiring the use of the affected arm, After the intervention, the results were obtained by applying a re-evaluation, where a remarkable improvement can be observed, giving results ranging between 6 - 11 points, giving a great improvement where it can be noted that a score 19 times lower than the initial interval and 31 times lower than the final interval of the scores obtained was obtained.

Degree of functionality in performing daily activities (initial assessment - final assessment)

Tabla 9.   User-rated epicondylitis test score - Activities of daily living

PATIENT NO.	DAILY ACTIVITIES	
	INITIAL EVALUATION	FINAL EVALUATION
Patient 1	24,0	8,0
Patient 2	24,0	8,0
Patient 3	28,0	6,0
Patient 4	26,0	9,0
Patient 5	24,0	15,0
Patient 6	27,0	11,0
Patient 7	23,0	9,0
Patient 8	23,0	9,0
Patient 9	24,0	7,0
Patient 10	25,0	12,0
Patient 11	28,0	13,0
Patient 12	22,0	10,0
Patient 13	23,0	13,0

| Patient 14 | 23,0 | 13,0 |
| Patient 15 | 32,0 | 9,0 |

Gráfico 8. Scoring User's epicondylitis elbow test - Daily activities

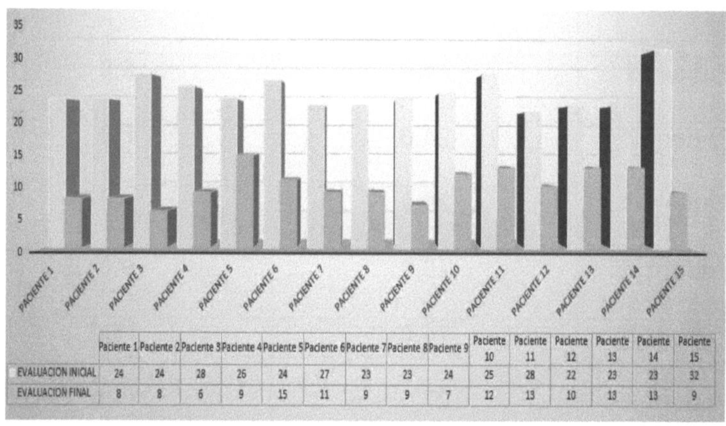

	Paciente 1	Paciente 2	Paciente 3	Paciente 4	Paciente 5	Paciente 6	Paciente 7	Paciente 8	Paciente 9	Paciente 10	Paciente 11	Paciente 12	Paciente 13	Paciente 14	Paciente 15
EVALUACION INICIAL	24	24	28	26	24	27	23	23	24	25	28	22	23	23	32
EVALUACION FINAL	8	8	6	9	15	11	9	9	7	12	13	10	13	13	9

Analysis and interpretation

In the present investigation in which the user-assessed epicondylitis test was used, an initial evaluation and a subsequent reevaluation of the patients was carried out. During the initial evaluation, scores were obtained that denoted an improvement in the users affected by elbow epicondylitis in the area of "daily activities", during the initial evaluation scores were obtained that ranged in intervals of 23 - 32 where the results showed that the patients had severe difficulty and disability in performing their daily activities, After the intervention, a reevaluation was applied, where a remarkable improvement can be observed, giving results ranging between 6 - 15 points, giving a great improvement where it can be noted that a score 17 times lower was obtained with respect to the initial interval and likewise 17 times lower with respect to the final interval of the first evaluation.

4.2   DISCUSSION

In the research of Galante José, in his research entitled "Tecartherapy in epicondylitis" at Fasta University, he shows that this method of thermotherapy resulted in the improvement of the symptomatology since it improves the blood flow, accelerating the healing process and helping to reduce pain in a time of 20 sessions. On the other hand, in this research with the title "Occupational therapy rehabilitation program for older adults with epicondylitis" shows a great progress through the therapeutic plan implemented individually to each patient with certain personalized routines with the placement of TENS and thermotherapy, that all the chosen patients had as a result an increase of articular range, decrease of pain and a greater grip in a lapse of 15 sessions per patient.

The results of this rehabilitation plan were notorious, since all showed improvement, each patient had a decrease in distress, increased grip action, increased range of motion and endurance.

In the work of Dr. Rosa Lopez, with the topic of work with its respective title as "Lateral epicondylitis. Therapeutic management" in Spain, gives as a result that the mobilization technique, which is to give movement in the joint passively by the therapist and active movements performed by the patient, which showed an increase in strength in the grip and decrease in pain, giving as a reference a noticeable increase in functionality. On my part, in the activities personalized to each patient, in the active exercises where resistance bands and weighted cylinders were used as an aid in a period of 15 sessions, where the patients performed them in the Hospital and an exercise regimen for their home, helped to obtain a considerable improvement in the increase of grip strength, increase of the range of motion, decrease of pain, increase of independence and resistance, where the patients had a greater range of motion, decrease of pain, increase of independence and resistance, where the patients who were registered in the research process with an evaluation where they gave results of low independence and high pain, culminated such sessions in the practice period, leaving the intervention plan to each one, helping them to continue improving progressively, giving them a good quality of life that they lost due to the pathology of epicondylitis.

Chapter V

CONCLUSIONS AND RECOMMENDATIONS

5.1 CONCLUSIONS

To identify the limitations of the patients chosen from the population with epicondylitis at the Teodoro Maldonado Carbo Hospital, in order to carry out evaluations and create a therapeutic rehabilitation program to improve their independence at home and in the work environment.

During the therapeutic activities and application of physical agents, motor or physical skills should be strengthened with the help of the intervention plan where it will be exercised day by day with a regimen of sessions adapted to the type of limitation.

Implement exercise routines such as flexion, extension, pronation and pronosupination together with TENS and thermotherapy, complying with the routines given to the patient every day in order to reduce pain in the affected area and increase the range of motion of the elbow.

The method by means of TENS, applied to patients, helped rehabilitation, benefiting in relieving pain and improving physical functions by means of electrical stimulation placed in the lateral area of the elbow affected by epicondylitis.

In the case of thermotherapy, it helps the area affected by epicondylitis, so that the pain in that region decreases, also helps to reduce stiffness, thus maximizing the functions of the person to perform work or daily life activities.

5.2 RECOMMENDATIONS

With respect to the pathology epicondylitis, and the research carried out, it is advisable for workers, when performing household chores and especially for older adults, to avoid repetitive movements and overexertion, as well as to avoid postures where the wrist remains in extension for a prolonged period of time. Do not pronate in a way that exerts great pressure on the tendons of the epicondyle.

In the case of the work environment, improving ergonomics would be based on your job, which by performing forced movements can generate epicondylitis, by improving ergonomics, that is, good posture, the risk of suffering this pathology drops considerably.

Given that epicondylitis is a pathology that most older adults acquire, it is advisable that both public and private institutions continue to intervene patients to raise awareness that it is a condition that, with the passage of time can produce serious functional limitations, and thus, create new intervention plans tailored to each person where they have positive results.

I recommend to my future colleagues in Occupational Therapy, to follow this study to implement this research, where there were beneficial results in all patients treated with the rehabilitation plan in epicondylitis for older adults.

BIBLIOGRAPHIC REFERENCES

1. López-Vidriero Tejedor R, López-Vidriero Tejedor E. Lateral epicondylitis. Therapeutic management. Rev Esp Artrosc Cir Articul [Internet]. September 2018 [cited May 29, 2023];25(2). Available from: https://fondoscience.com/reaca/vol25-fasc2-num63/fs1711059-epicondilitis-lateral-manejo-terapeutico

Jiménez Solís F, Arboine Ciphas M, Solórzano Herra S, Jiménez Solís F, Arboine Ciphas M, Solórzano Herra S. Epicondylitis: Literature review from a medicolegal perspective. Med Leg Costa Rica. March 2021;38(1):80-8.

Moros Marco S, Asenjo Gismero CV, Del Monte Bello G, Paniagua González A, Jiménez Fermín M, Pintado López G, et al. Epicondylitis (lateral elbow tendinopathy): diagnostic strategies and classification. Rev Esp Artrosc Cir Articul [Internet]. December 2020 [cited May 29, 2023];27(4). Available from: https://fondoscience.com/reaca/vol27-fasc4-num70/fs2001007-epicondilitis-tendinopatia-lateral-codo

4. Sánchez NM. What do we know about tennis elbow or lateral epicondylalgia? [Internet]. KHINN Center. 2022 [cited 2023 May 29, 2023]. Available from: https://www.khinncenter.com/codo-de-tenista/

5. Pina JC, Calvo MG. Prevention and treatment of "tennis elbow" injury, epicondylitis, in adult athletes: a systematic review.

6. Labrada Rodríguez YH, Escribano Rodríguez M, Hernández Pretel NI, Arribas Manzanal PD, López de Lacey EM, Garvín Ocampos L, et al. Mid-term results of piezoelectric shock wave therapy in lateral epicondylitis. Correo Científico Méd. March 2020;24(1):73-87.

7. Nivelo RV Boxes. Treatment of lateral epicondylitis in adults. Univ Católica Cuenca [Internet]. 2022 [cited 2023 June 2, 2023]; Available from: https://dspace.ucacue.edu.ec/handle/ucacue/13070

8. Rodríguez Monterde I, Méndez Sánchez J. Conservative treatment plan in the pathology of lateral epicondylitis of the elbow. 2022 [cited June 2, 2023]; Available from: https://riull.ull.es/xmlui/handle/915/28607

Torres ELN, Torres ESN, Díaz AAN, Barroso FR, Otazo EIL. Physical agents and eccentric training in humeral epicondylitis. Arch Hosp Univ Gen Calixto Garcia. Aug 7, 2019;7(2):209-21.

10. Pimentel GC, Fernández AL, Jara JF, Galán SL, Villarreal EP. Review of the most frequent sports injuries in the practice of paddle tennis. Seram [Internet]. May 26, 2022 [cited June 2, 2023];1(1). Available from: https://www.piper.espacio-seram.com/index.php/seram/article/view/9263

11.   Ramirez Salvany G. Mulligan technique for the physiotherapeutic treatment of epicondylitis: systematic review. 2022 [cited 2022 June 2, 2023]; Available from: https://repositori.tecnocampus.cat/handle/20.500.12367/2048

12.   Planas Lara AE, Docun Lecumberri M, Tomás Royo JA. Application aid for the assessment of professional epicondylitis and epicondylitis epitrocleitis. In: Actas III Congreso Prevencionar 2021: Ciencia, conocimiento y transferencia, 2022, ISBN 978-84-09-40683-8, pp 79-87 [Internet]. Seguridad y Bienestar Laboral S.L.; 2022 [cited 2023 June 2]. p. 79-87. Available from: https://dialnet.unirioja.es/servlet/articulo?codigo=8409631

13.   López-Brito J, Moreno-Jiménez RM, Regal-Ramos RJ, López-Brito J, Moreno-Jiménez RM, Regal-Ramos RJ. Descriptive analysis of permanent disability records due to epicondylitis in food industry workers. Med Segur Trab. June 2021;67(263):128-54.

14.   Object object. Efficacy of electrotherapy methods in the treatment of lateral epicondylitis taking into account pain and grip strength. Systematic review. [cited June 13, 2023]; Available from: https://core.ac.uk/reader/324149140

15.   López-Vidriero Tejedor R, López-Vidriero Tejedor E. Lateral epicondylitis. Therapeutic management. Rev Esp Artrosc Cir Articul [Internet]. September 2018 [cited June 12, 2023];25(2). Available from: https://fondoscience.com/reaca/vol25-fasc2-num63/fs1711059-epicondilitis-lateral-manejo-terapeutico

Valderrama Alfonso AF, Salazar Díaz CM. Quantitative analysis of percutaneous neuromodulation therapy in the treatment of lateral epicondylitis from the analysis of the muscle pattern observed with multichannel semg signals. 2021 [cited June 16, 2023]; Available from: https://repositorio.unbosque.edu.co/handle/20.500.12495/6946

Moreno B, Muñoz M, Cuellar J, Domancic S, Villanueva J, Moreno B, et al. Systematic reviews: definition and basic notions. Rev Clinica Periodoncia Implantol Rehabil Oral. December 2018;11(3):184-6.

18.   Merino Alvarez FJ. Effects of myofascial release of the biceps brachii and tens on elbow pain, hand prehensile strength and upper extremity functionality in women with chronic lateral epicondylalgia symptomatology. 2018 [cited July 12, 2023]; Available from: https://repositorio.unab.cl/xmlui/handle/ria/21759

19.   Gonzalez S. Benefits of thermotherapy in functional recovery. 2018;

20.   Vega Yepez VDR. PREVALENCE OF SKELETAL MUSCLE DISEASES ASSOCIATED WITH WORK ACTIVITY IN THE WORKERS OF THE HEALTH SYSTEMS OF THE UNIVERSITY SAN FRANCISCO DE QUITO - SIME [Internet] [master thesis]. Quito, Ecuador: Universidad Tecnológica

Israel; 2022 [cited July 16, 2023]. Available from:
http://repositorio.uisrael.edu.ec/handle/47000/3069

Annexes

Annex 1. Data collection form

BARTHEL'S INDEX
BASIC ACTIVITIES OF DAILY LIVING
Patient:
Age: Sex: Occupation: Diagnosis:

Parameter	Patient situation	Score
Eat	Totally dependent	
	Need help cutting food	
	Dependent	
Wash	Independent: in and out of the bathroom	
	Dependent	
Dress	Independent: able to put on and take off clothes	
	Need help	
	Dependent	
Using the toilet	Independent	
	Need help	
	Dependent	
Go to	Stand-alone to go to the couch to bed	
	Need help	
	Dependent	

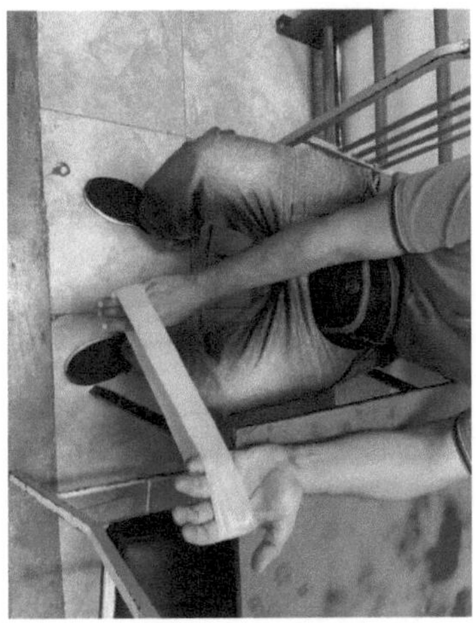

Supination exercise with an elastic band in a patient with epicondylitis.

ANNEX 3. PRONATION EXERCISE WITH ELASTIC BAND.

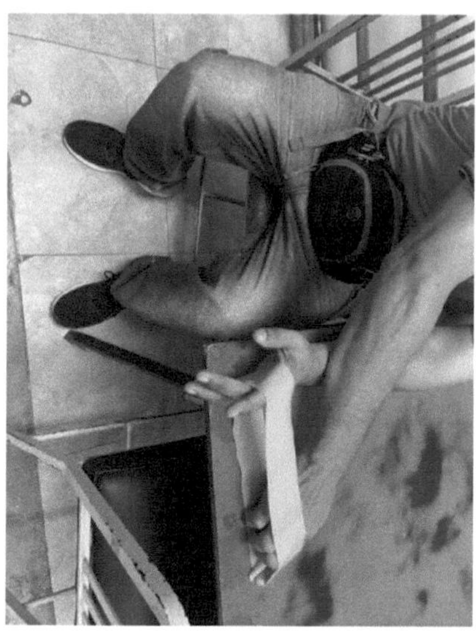

Pronation exercise with an elastic band in a patient with epicondylitis.

APPENDIX 4. EPICONDYLAR STRETCHING EXERCISE.

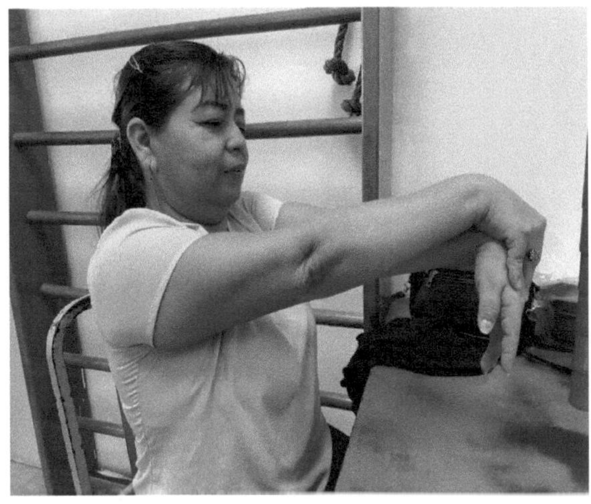

Epicondylar stretching exercise in a patient with epicondylitis.

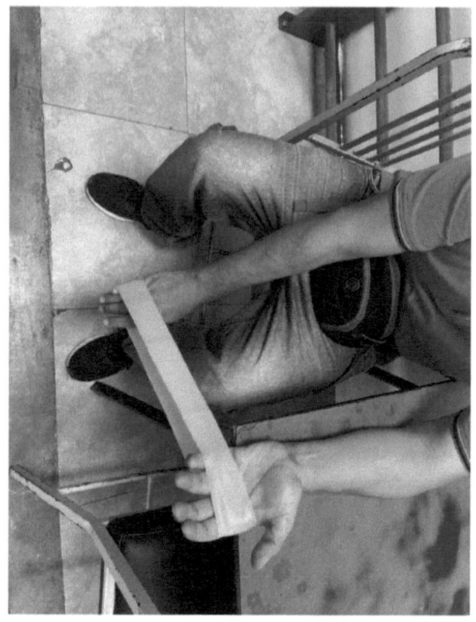

Wrist flexion exercise with an elastic band in a patient with epicondylitis.

APPENDIX 6. WRIST EXTENSION EXERCISE WITH AN ELASTIC BAND

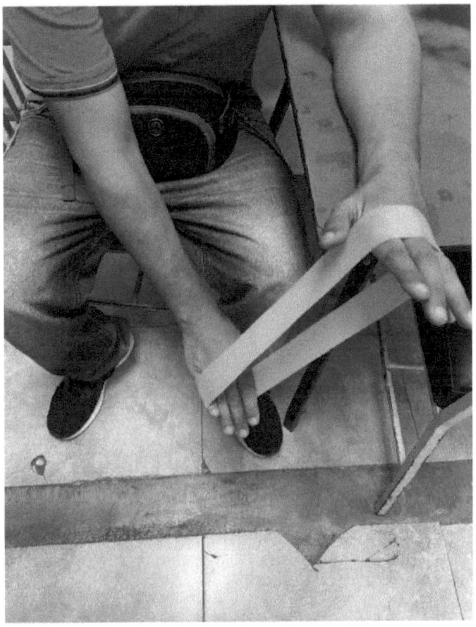

Wrist extension exercise with an elastic band in a patient with epicondylitis.

ANNEX 7. PRONOSUPINATION EXERCISE WITH CYLINDER.

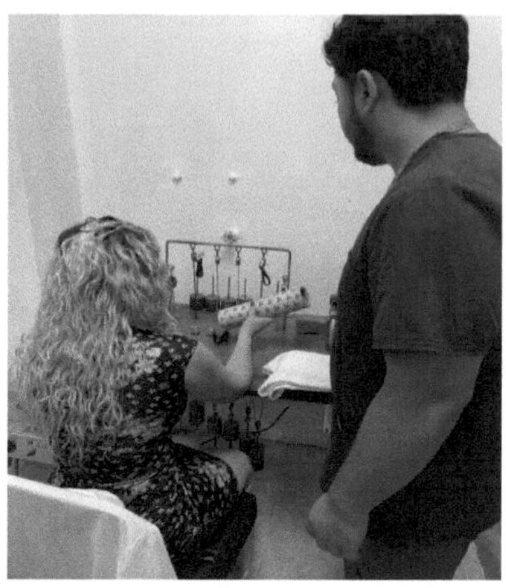

Pronosupination exercise with cylinder in a patient with epicondylitis.

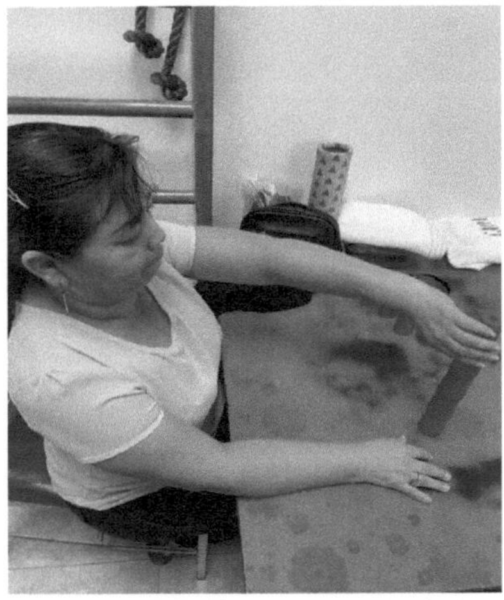

Pronosupination exercise with cones in a patient with epicondylitis.

ANNEX 9. PRONATION EXERCISE WITH WEIGHTS

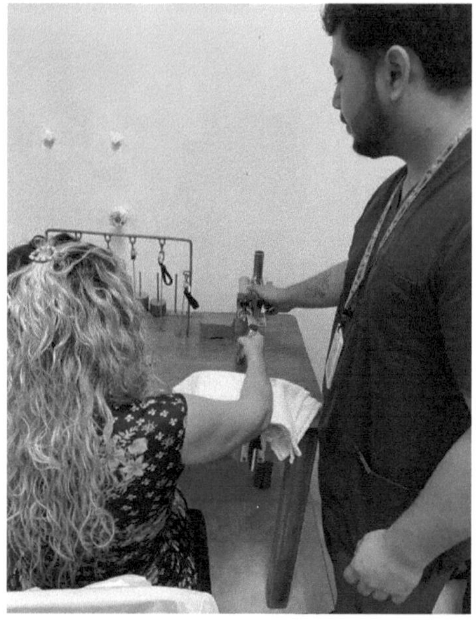

Pronation exercise with weights in a patient with epicondylitis.

ANNEX 10. APPLICATION OF TENS

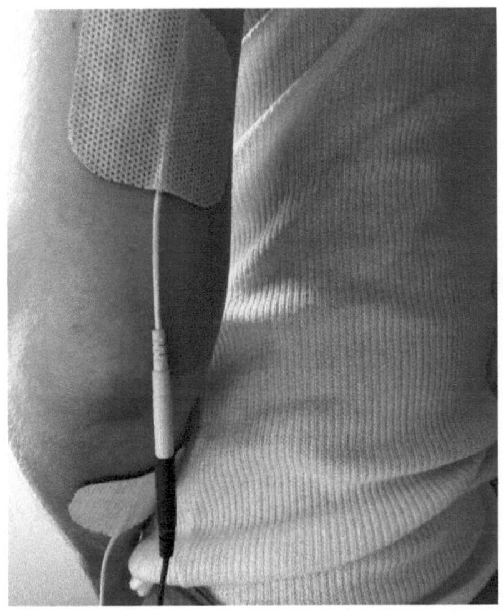

TENS application in patient with epicondylitis.

ANNEX 11. THERMOTHERAPY

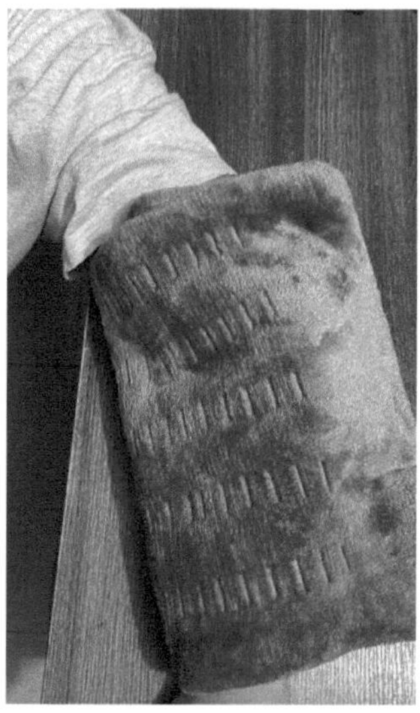

Application of thermotherapy in patient with epicondylitis.

ANNEX 12. EVALUATION

BARTHEL'S INDEX
BASIC ACTIVITIES OF DAILY LIVING
Patient: Oyague
Age: 61 Sex: Female Occupation: Dentist Diagnosis: Epicondylitis

Parameter	Patient situation	Score
Eat	Totally dependent	10,0
	Need help cutting food	5,0
	Dependent	0,0
Wash	Independent: in and out of the bathroom	5,0
	Dependent	0,0
Dress	Independent: able to put on and take off clothes	10,0
	Need help	5,0
	Dependent	0,0
Using the toilet	Independent	10,0
	Need help	5,0
	Dependent	0,0
Go to	Stand-alone to go to the couch to bed	10,0
	Need help	5,0
	Dependent	0,0

Patient: Gloria
Age: 63 Sex: Female Occupation: Secretary Diagnosis: Epicondylitis

Parameter	Patient situation	Score
Eat	Totally dependent	10,0
	Need help cutting food	5,0
	Dependent	0,0
Wash	Independent: in and out of the bathroom	5,0
	Dependent	0,0
Dress	Independent: able to put on and take off clothes	10,0
	Need help	5,0
	Dependent	0,0
Using the toilet	Independent	10,0
	Need help	5,0
	Dependent	0,0
Go to	Stand-alone to go to the couch to bed	10,0
	Need help	5,0
	Dependent	0,0

Patient: Juana

Age: 67 Sex: Female Occupation: Assistant Diagnosis: Epicondylitis

Parameter	Patient situation	Score
Eat	Totally dependent	10,0
	Need help cutting food	5,0
	Dependent	0,0
Wash	Independent: in and out of the bathroom	5,0
	Dependent	0,0
Dress	Independent: able to put on and take off clothes	10,0
	Need help	5,0
	Dependent	0,0
Using the toilet	Independent	10,0
	Need help	5,0
	Dependent	0,0
Go to	Stand-alone to go to the couch to bed	10,0
	Need help	5,0
	Dependent	0,0

Patient: Diana

Age: 71 Sex: Female Occupation: Homemaker Diagnosis: Epicondylitis

Parameter	Patient situation	Score
Eat	Totally dependent	10,0
	Need help cutting food	5,0
	Dependent	0,0
Wash	Independent: in and out of the bathroom	5,0
	Dependent	0,0
Dress	Independent: able to put on and take off clothes	10,0
	Need help	5,0
	Dependent	0,0
Using the toilet	Independent	10,0
	Need help	5,0
	Dependent	0,0
Go to	Stand-alone to go to the couch to bed	10,0
	Need help	5,0
	Dependent	0,0

Patient: Vilma
Age: 67 Sex: Female Occupation: Homemaker Diagnosis: Epicondylitis

Parameter	Patient situation	Score
Eat	Totally dependent	10,0
	Need help cutting food	5,0
	Dependent	0,0
Wash	Independent: in and out of the bathroom	5,0
	Dependent	0,0
Dress	Independent: able to put on and take off clothes	10,0
	Need help	5,0
	Dependent	0,0
Using the toilet	Independent	10,0
	Need help	5,0
	Dependent	0,0
Go to	Stand-alone to go to the couch to bed	10,0
	Need help	5,0
	Dependent	0,0

Patient: Melany
Age: 66 Sex: Female Occupation: Human Resources Diagnosis: Epicondylitis

Parameter	Patient situation	Score
Eat	Totally dependent	10,0
	Need help cutting food	5,0
	Dependent	0,0
Wash	Independent: in and out of the bathroom	5,0
	Dependent	0,0
Dress	Independent: able to put on and take off clothes	10,0
	Need help	5,0
	Dependent	0,0
Using the toilet	Independent	10,0
	Need help	5,0
	Dependent	0,0
Go to	Stand-alone to go to the couch to bed	10,0
	Need help	5,0
	Dependent	0,0

Patient: Marlon

Age: 73 Sex: Male Occupation: Cook Diagnosis: Epicondylitis

Parameter	Patient situation	Score
Eat	Totally dependent	10,0
	Need help cutting food	5,0
	Dependent	0,0
Wash	Independent: in and out of the bathroom	5,0
	Dependent	0,0
Dress	Independent: able to put on and take off clothes	10,0
	Need help	5,0
	Dependent	0,0
Using the toilet	Independent	10,0
	Need help	5,0
	Dependent	0,0
Go to	Stand-alone to go to the couch to bed	10,0
	Need help	5,0
	Dependent	0,0

Patient: Xavier

Age: 68 Sex: Male Occupation: Goalkeeper Diagnosis: Epicondylitis

Parameter	Patient situation	Score
Eat	Totally dependent	10,0
	Need help cutting food	5,0
	Dependent	0,0
Wash	Independent: in and out of the bathroom	5,0
	Dependent	0,0
Dress	Independent: able to put on and take off clothes	10,0
	Need help	5,0
	Dependent	0,0
Using the toilet	Independent	10,0
	Need help	5,0
	Dependent	0,0
Go to	Stand-alone to go to the couch to bed	10,0
	Need help	5,0
	Dependent	0,0

Patient: Susan

Age: 76 Sex: Female Occupation: Homemaker Diagnosis: Epicondylitis

Parameter	Patient situation	Score
Eat	Totally dependent	10,0
	Need help cutting food	5,0
	Dependent	0,0
Wash	Independent: in and out of the bathroom	5,0
	Dependent	0,0
Dress	Independent: able to put on and take off clothes	10,0
	Need help	5,0
	Dependent	0,0
Using the toilet	Independent	10,0
	Need help	5,0
	Dependent	0,0
Go to	Stand-alone to go to the couch to bed	10,0
	Need help	5,0
	Dependent	0,0

Patient: Mauricio

Age: 69 Sex: Male Occupation: Not working Diagnosis: Epicondylitis

Parameter	Patient situation	Score
Eat	Totally dependent	10,0
	Need help cutting food	5,0
	Dependent	0,0
Wash	Independent: in and out of the bathroom	5,0
	Dependent	0,0
Dress	Independent: able to put on and take off clothes	10,0
	Need help	5,0
	Dependent	0,0
Using the toilet	Independent	10,0
	Need help	5,0
	Dependent	0,0
Go to	Stand-alone to go to the couch to bed	10,0
	Need help	5,0
	Dependent	0,0

Patient: Milena

Age: 67 Sex: Female Occupation: Accountant Diagnosis: Epicondylitis

Parameter	Patient situation	Score
Eat	Totally dependent	10,0
	Need help cutting food	5,0
	Dependent	0,0
Wash	Independent: in and out of the bathroom	5,0
	Dependent	0,0
Dress	Independent: able to put on and take off clothes	10,0
	Need help	5,0
	Dependent	0,0
Using the toilet	Independent	10,0
	Need help	5,0
	Dependent	0,0
Go to	Stand-alone to go to the couch to bed	10,0
	Need help	5,0
	Dependent	0,0

Patient: Alejandro

Age: 61 Sex: Male Occupation: Machine Operator Diagnosis: Epicondylitis

Parameter	Patient situation	Score
Eat	Totally dependent	10,0
	Need help cutting food	5,0
	Dependent	0,0
Wash	Independent: in and out of the bathroom	5,0
	Dependent	0,0
Dress	Independent: able to put on and take off clothes	10,0
	Need help	5,0
	Dependent	0,0
Using the toilet	Independent	10,0
	Need help	5,0
	Dependent	0,0
Go to	Stand-alone to go to the couch to bed	10,0
	Need help	5,0
	Dependent	0,0

Patient: Ana

Age: 82 Sex: Female Occupation: Homemaker Diagnosis: Epicondylitis

Parameter	Patient situation	Score
Eat	Totally dependent	10,0
	Need help cutting food	5,0
	Dependent	0,0
Wash	Independent: in and out of the bathroom	5,0
	Dependent	0,0
Dress	Independent: able to put on and take off clothes	10,0
	Need help	5,0
	Dependent	0,0
Using the toilet	Independent	10,0
	Need help	5,0
	Dependent	0,0
Go to	Stand-alone to go to the couch to bed	10,0
	Need help	5,0
	Dependent	0,0

ANNEX 13. REVALUATION

Patient: Oyague
Age: 61 Sex: Female Occupation: Dentist Diagnosis: Epicondylitis

Parameter	Patient situation	Score
Eat	Totally dependent	10,0
	Need help cutting food	5,0
	Dependent	0,0
Wash	Independent: in and out of the bathroom	5,0
	Dependent	0,0
Dress	Independent: able to put on and take off clothes	10,0
	Need help	5,0
	Dependent	0,0
Using the toilet	Independent	10,0
	Need help	5,0
	Dependent	0,0
Go to	Stand-alone to go to the couch to bed	10,0
	Need help	5,0
	Dependent	0,0

Patient: Gloria
Age: 63 Sex: Female Occupation: Secretary Diagnosis: Epicondylitis

Parameter	Patient situation	Score
Eat	Totally dependent	10,0
	Need help cutting food	5,0
	Dependent	0,0
Wash	Independent: in and out of the bathroom	5,0
	Dependent	0,0
Dress	Independent: capable of putting on and taking off clothes	10,0
	Need help	5,0
	Dependent	0,0
Using the toilet	Independent	10,0
	Need help	5,0
	Dependent	0,0
Go to	Stand-alone to go to the couch to bed	10,0
	Need help	5,0
	Dependent	0,0

Patient: Juana
Age: 67 Sex: Female Occupation: Assistant Diagnosis: Epicondylitis

Parameter	Patient situation	Score
Eat	Totally dependent	10,0
	Need help cutting food	5,0
	Dependent	0,0
Wash	Independent: in and out of the bathroom	5,0
	Dependent	0,0
Dress	Independent: able to put on and take off clothes	10,0
	Need help	5,0
	Dependent	0,0
Using the toilet	Independent	10,0
	Need help	5,0
	Dependent	0,0
Go to	Stand-alone to go to the couch to bed	10,0
	Need help	5,0
	Dependent	0,0

Patient: Diana
Age: 71 Sex: Female Occupation: Homemaker Diagnosis: Epicondylitis

Parameter	Patient situation	Score
Eat	Totally dependent	10,0
	Need help cutting food	5,0
	Dependent	0,0
Wash	Independent: in and out of the bathroom	5,0
	Dependent	0,0
Dress	Independent: able to put on and take off clothes	10,0
	Need help	5,0
	Dependent	0,0
Using the toilet	Independent	10,0
	Need help	5,0
	Dependent	0,0
Go to	Stand-alone to go to the couch to bed	10,0
	Need help	5,0
	Dependent	0,0

Patient: Vilma

Age: 67 Sex: Female Occupation: Homemaker Diagnosis: Epicondylitis

Parameter	Patient situation	Score
Eat	Totally dependent	10,0
	Need help cutting food	5,0
	Dependent	0,0
Wash	Independent: in and out of the bathroom	5,0
	Dependent	0,0
Dress	Independent: able to put on and take off clothes	10,0
	Need help	5,0
	Dependent	0,0
Using the toilet	Independent	10,0
	Need help	5,0
	Dependent	0,0
Go to	Stand-alone to go to the couch to bed	10,0
	Need help	5,0
	Dependent	0,0

Patient: Melany

Age: 66 Sex: Female Occupation: Human Resources Diagnosis: Epicondylitis

Parameter	Patient situation	Score
Eat	Totally dependent	10,0
	Need help cutting food	5,0
	Dependent	0,0
Wash	Independent: in and out of the bathroom	5,0
	Dependent	0,0
Dress	Independent: able to put on and take off clothes	10,0
	Need help	5,0
	Dependent	0,0
Using the toilet	Independent	10,0
	Need help	5,0
	Dependent	0,0
Go to	Stand-alone to go to the couch to bed	10,0
	Need help	5,0
	Dependent	0,0

Patient: Marlon

Age: 73 Sex: Male Occupation: Cook Diagnosis: Epicondylitis

Parameter	Patient situation	Score
Eat	Totally dependent	10,0
	Need help cutting food	5,0
	Dependent	0,0
Wash	Independent: in and out of the bathroom	5,0
	Dependent	0,0
Dress	Independent: able to put on and take off clothes	10,0
	Need help	5,0
	Dependent	0,0
Using the toilet	Independent	10,0
	Need help	5,0
	Dependent	0,0
Go to	Stand-alone to go to the couch to bed	10,0
	Need help	5,0
	Dependent	0,0

Patient: Xavier

Age: 68 Sex: Male Occupation: Goalkeeper Diagnosis: Epicondylitis

Parameter	Patient situation	Score
Eat	Totally dependent	10,0
	Need help cutting food	5,0
	Dependent	0,0
Wash	Independent: in and out of the bathroom	5,0
	Dependent	0,0
Dress	Independent: able to put on and take off clothes	10,0
	Need help	5,0
	Dependent	0,0
Using the toilet	Independent	10,0
	Need help	5,0
	Dependent	0,0
Go to	Stand-alone to go to the couch to bed	10,0
	Need help	5,0
	Dependent	0,0

Patient: Susan

Age: 76 Sex: Female Occupation: Homemaker Diagnosis: Epicondylitis

Parameter	Patient situation	Score
Eat	Totally dependent	10,0
	Need help cutting food	5,0
	Dependent	0,0
Wash	Independent: in and out of the bathroom	5,0
	Dependent	0,0
Dress	Independent: able to put on and take off clothes	10,0
	Need help	5,0
	Dependent	0,0
Using the toilet	Independent	10,0
	Need help	5,0
	Dependent	0,0
Go to	Stand-alone to go to the couch to bed	10,0
	Need help	5,0
	Dependent	0,0

Patient: Mauricio

Age: 69 Sex: Male Occupation: Not working Diagnosis: Epicondylitis

Parameter	Patient situation	Score
Eat	Totally dependent	10,0
	Need help cutting food	5,0
	Dependent	0,0
Wash	Independent: in and out of the bathroom	5,0
	Dependent	0,0
Dress	Independent: capable of putting on and taking off clothes	10,0
	Need help	5,0
	Dependent	0,0
Using the toilet	Independent	10,0
	Need help	5,0
	Dependent	0,0
Go to	Independent to go to the couch to bed	10,0
	Need help	5,0
	Dependent	0,0

Patient: Milena

Age: 67 Sex: Female Occupation: Accountant Diagnosis: Epicondylitis

Parameter	Patient situation	Score
Eat	Totally dependent	10,0
	Need help cutting food	5,0
	Dependent	0,0
Wash	Independent: in and out of the bathroom	5,0
	Dependent	0,0
Dress	Independent: able to put on and take off clothes	10,0
	Need help	5,0
	Dependent	0,0
Using the toilet	Independent	10,0
	Need help	5,0
	Dependent	0,0
Go to	Stand-alone to go to the couch to bed	10,0
	Need help	5,0
	Dependent	0,0

Patient: Alejandro

Age: 61 Sex: Male Occupation: Machine Operator Diagnosis: Epicondylitis

Parameter	Patient situation	Score
Eat	Totally dependent	10,0
	Need help cutting food	5,0
	Dependent	0,0
Wash	Independent: in and out of the bathroom	5,0
	Dependent	0,0
Dress	Independent: able to put on and take off clothes	10,0
	Need help	5,0
	Dependent	0,0
Using the toilet	Independent	10,0
	Need help	5,0
	Dependent	0,0
Go to	Stand-alone to go to the couch to bed	10,0
	Need help	5,0
	Dependent	0,0

Patient: Ana

Age: 82 Sex: Female Occupation: Homemaker Diagnosis: Epicondylitis

Parameter	Patient situation	Score
Eat	Totally dependent	10,0
	Need help cutting food	5,0
	Dependent	0,0
Wash	Independent: in and out of the bathroom	5,0
	Dependent	0,0
Dress	Independent: able to put on and take off clothes	10,0
	Need help	5,0
	Dependent	0,0
Using the toilet	Independent	10,0
	Need help	5,0
	Dependent	0,0
Go to	Stand-alone to go to the couch to bed	10,0
	Need help	5,0
	Dependent	0,0

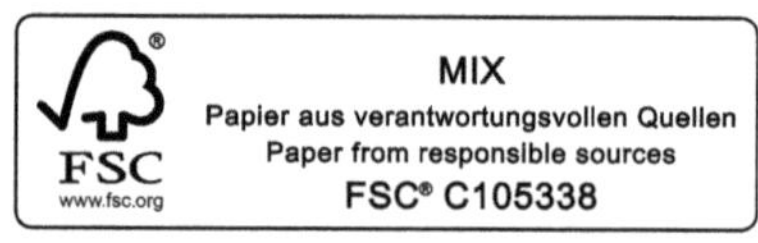

Printed by Books on Demand GmbH, Norderstedt / Germany